# Might C  Vs.  Cancer

I0500366

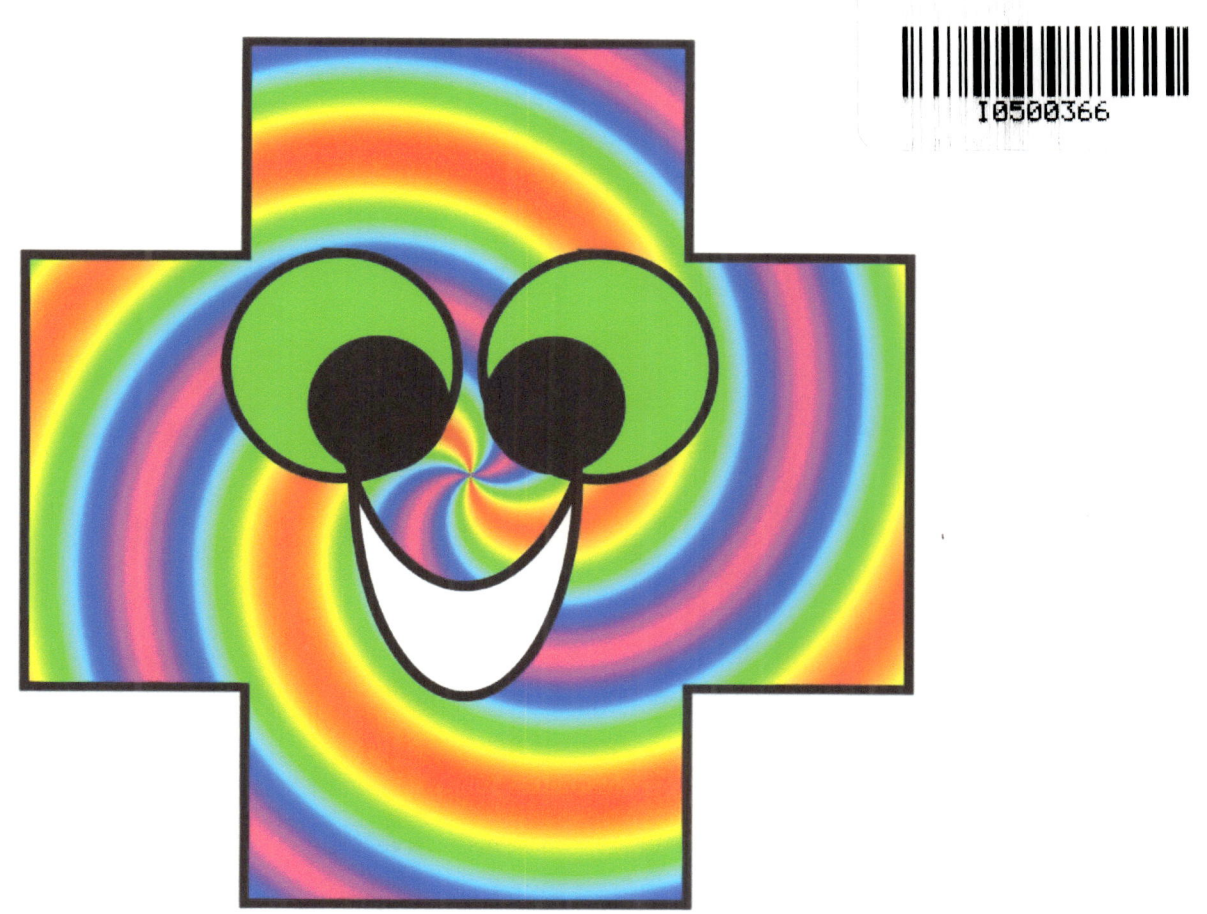

Written by:  Sunny Schellinger Krowski

ISBN-10: 1515150364
ISBN-13: 978-1515150367

Printed in the United States of America

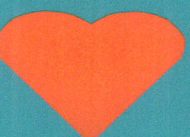 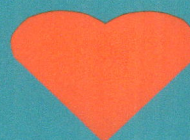

# Dedication

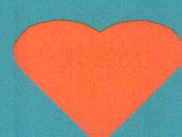 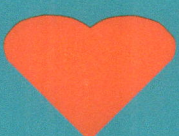

I wrote this book to help all of the children in my life who needed to understand my battle. I dedicate this book to each of them. They know who they are, they know how special they are to me and they know I live for them.

Love,

Mom, Aunt Sunny, Ms. Sunny

# ACKNOWLEDGMENTS

JAMES FOR HELPING ME DESIGN ALL OF THE FUN CHARACTERS IN THE BOOK.  MY HUSBAND, WHO HAS ALWAYS GIVEN ME UNWAVERING LOVE AND SUPPORT, BECAUSE OF HIM, I ALWAYS FEEL BEAUTIFUL.  MY FAMILY FOR ALWAYS BELIEVING IN ME. MY SISTER, DEBBIE, FOR PUSHING ME TO GET MY BOOK PUBLISHED.  MY COUSIN, VIRGINIA, FOR ALL OF HER HELP GETTING THE BOOK PUBLISHED.  JOSEPH AND JULIA FOR SURVIVING INSPITE OF MY ABSENCE.  MY CHURCH, PARK HILL PRESBYTERIAN CHURCH, FOR LOVING AND SUPPORTING ME THROUGHOUT MY JOURNEY.  DR. JAMES HAGANS, III FOR FINDING MY CANCER AND GIVING ME SUPPORT TO MAKE THE RIGHT DECISIONS REGUARDING MY CARE AND FOR LETTING ME USE HIS PICTURE IN THE BOOK.  DR. BALTZ AND ALL OF HIS STAFF, FOR GIVING ME THE BEST CARE AVAILABLE.

The child asked the parent, "What is cancer?"

The parent answered, "That is a hard question. Here is the best way I can explain it to you."

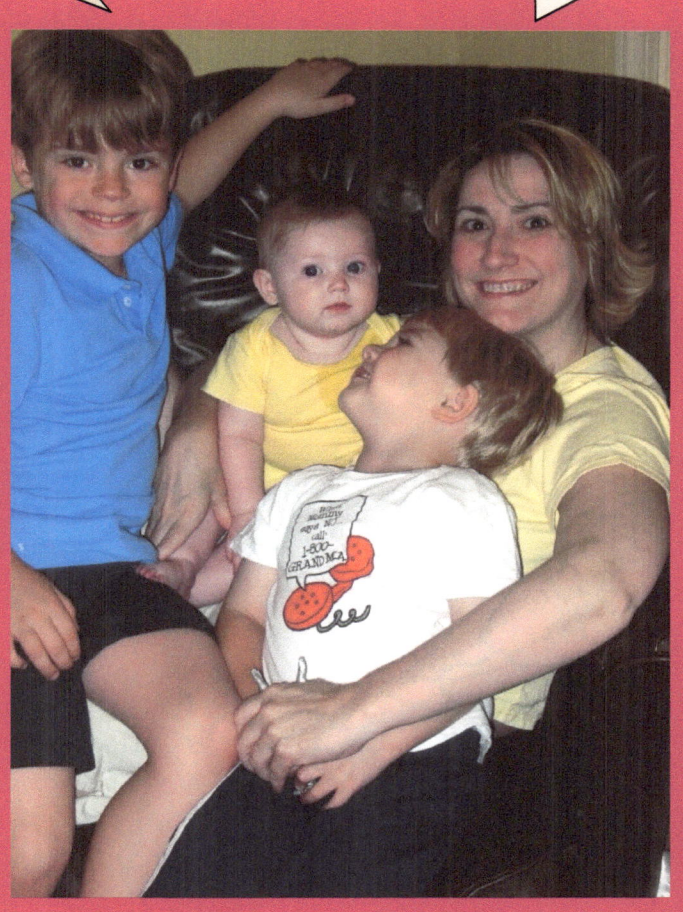

Our bodies are made up of cells.

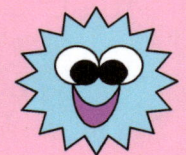

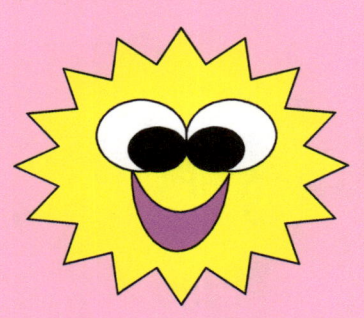

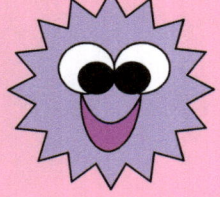

These cells are good cells.

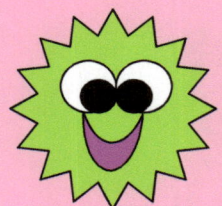

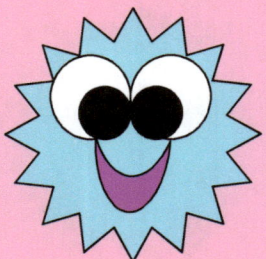

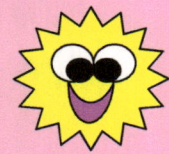

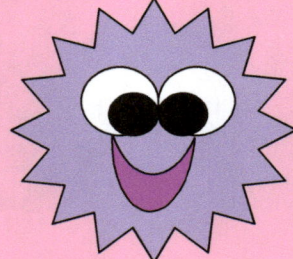

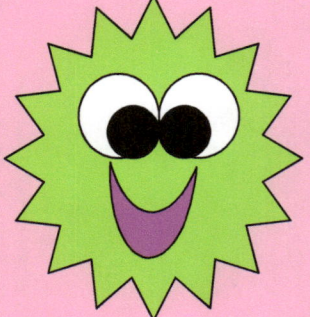

Healthy people
sometimes have
some bad cells.

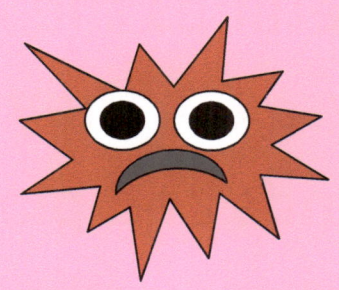

But, the body keeps the bad cells away from each
other and the good cells try to play nice with the
bad cells to teach them how to be good.

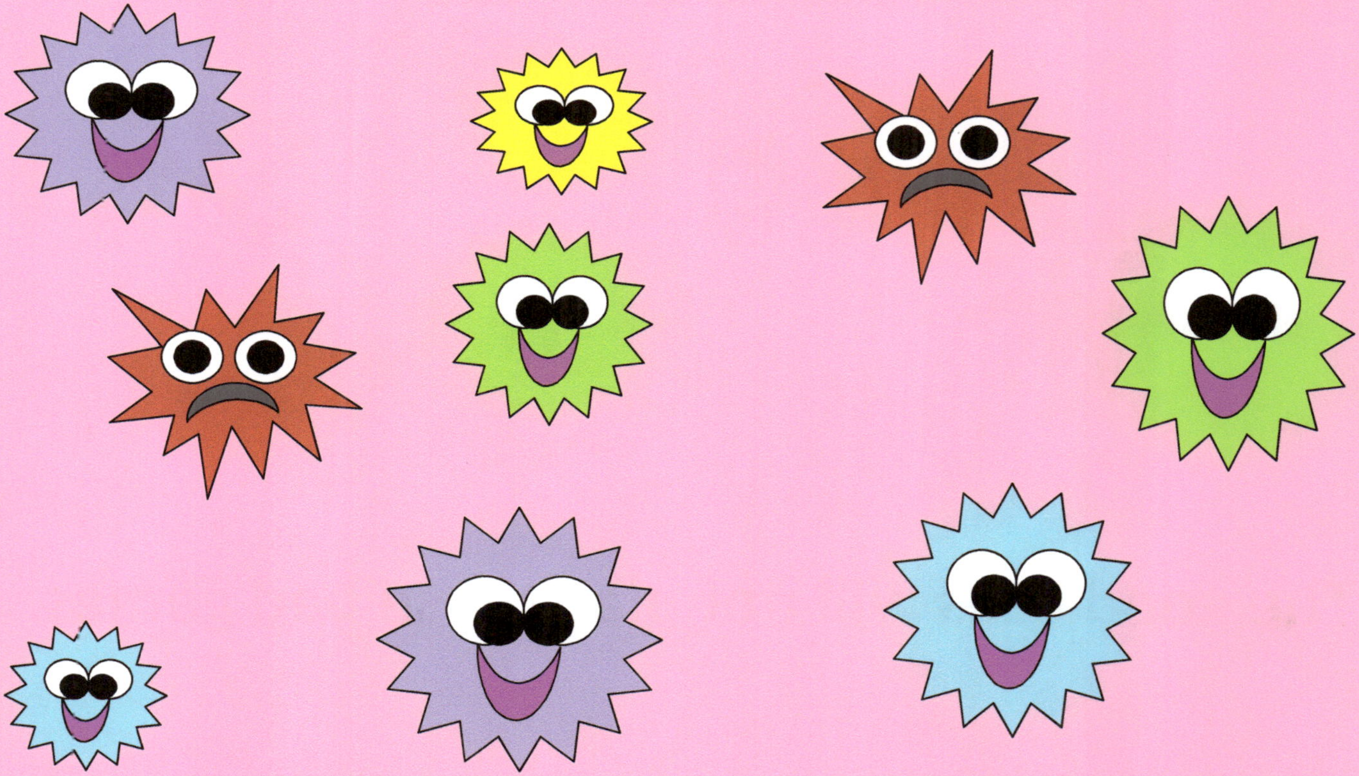

But, sometimes the bad cells want to do bad things.  So, they go looking for cells to be friends and play bad games with.

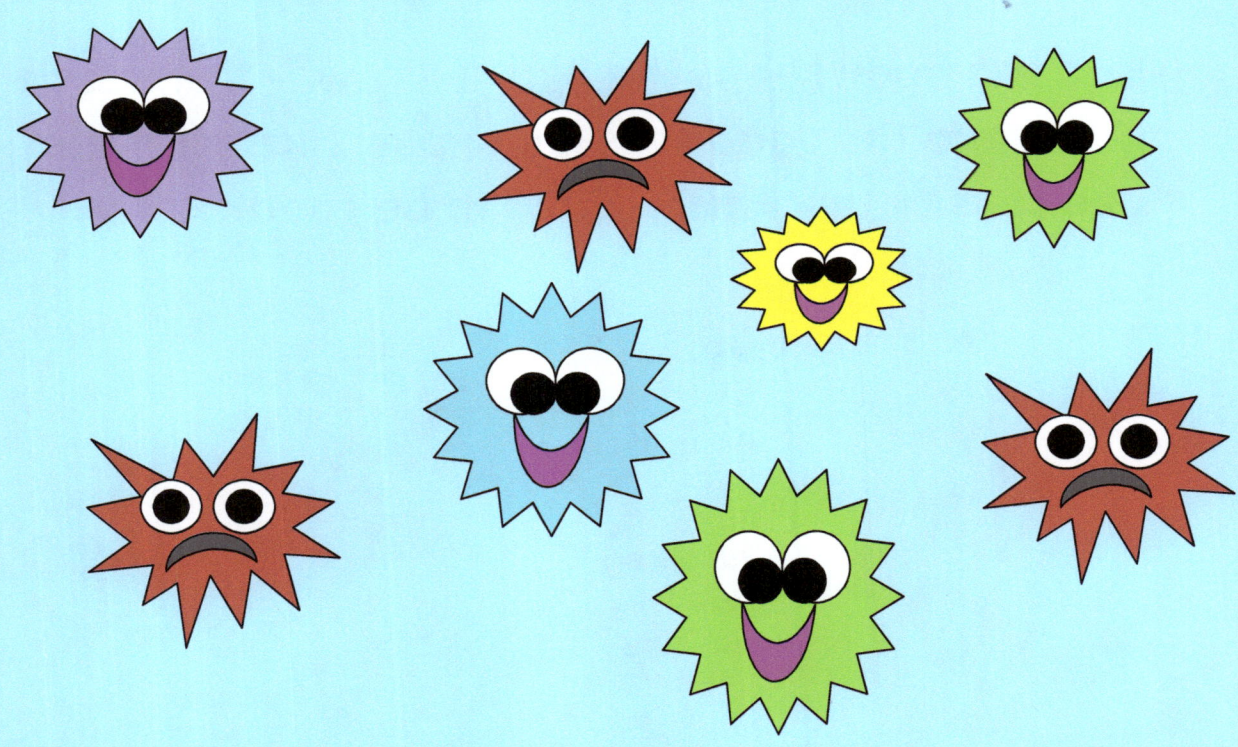

The good cells will not play these bad games.

If the bad cells find more bad cells, they make a group of bad cells and call themselves a "tumor".

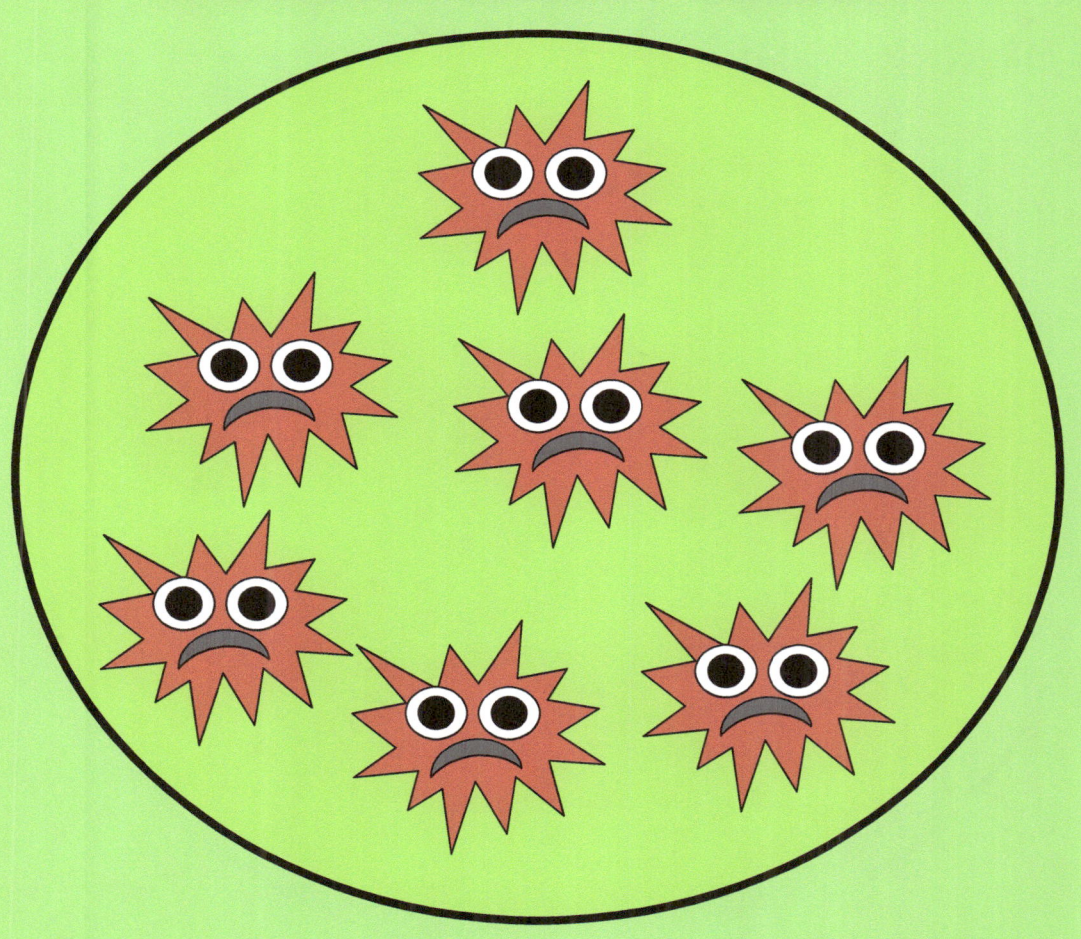

The tumor gang may stay together and just play their bad games as a group of friends.

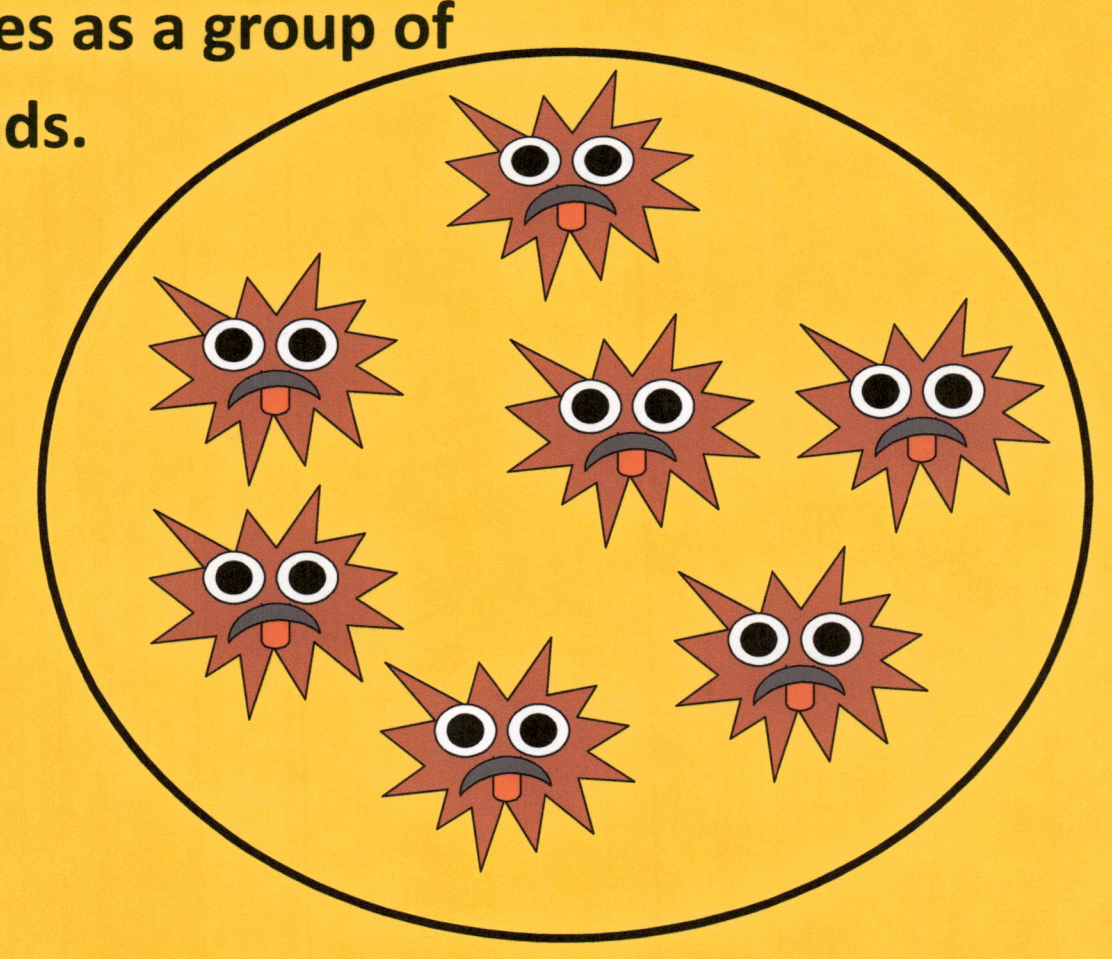

Tumor gangs play really hard.  So, they need lots of food.   They search for any food that is eaten.  They want to become stronger.

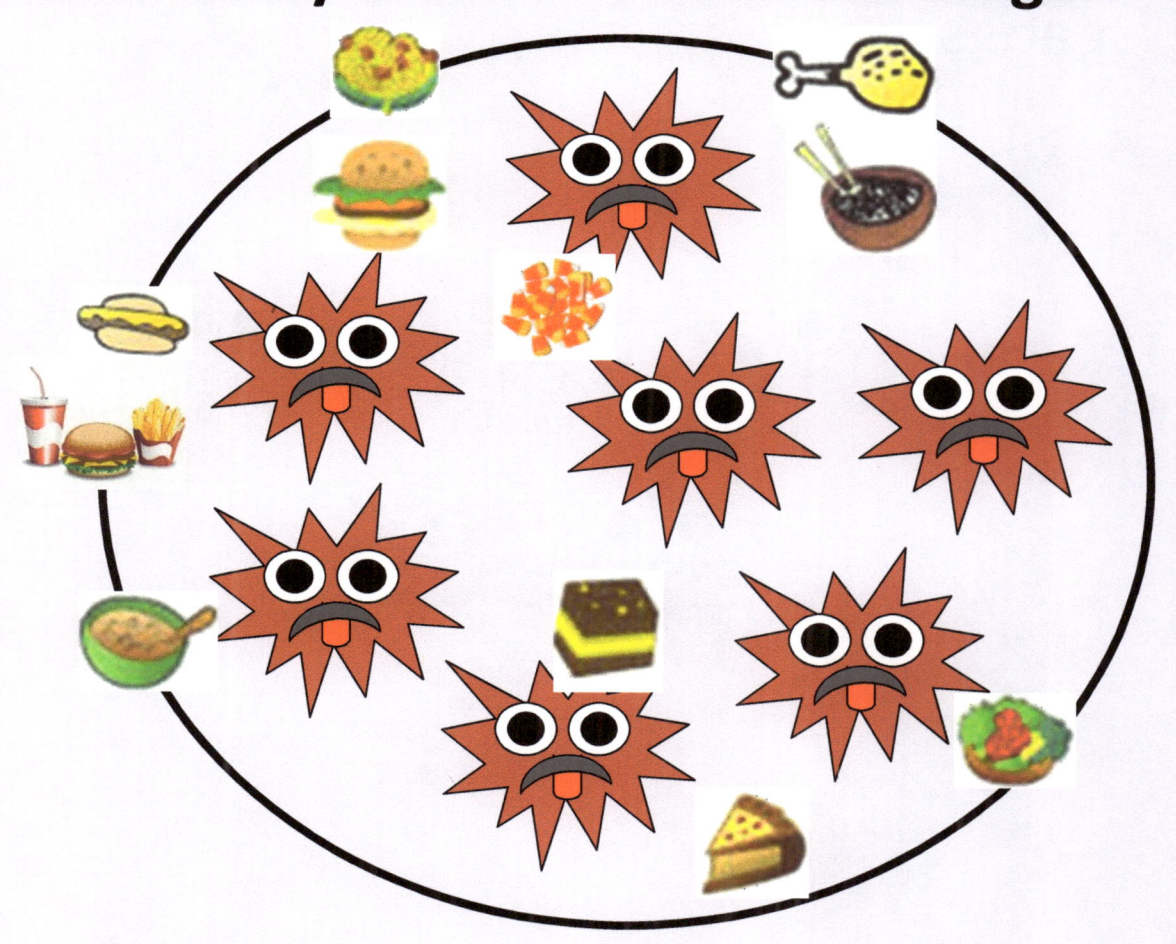

While they get stronger, the body gets weaker.  Sometimes they get so strong that they become "Cancer" gangs.

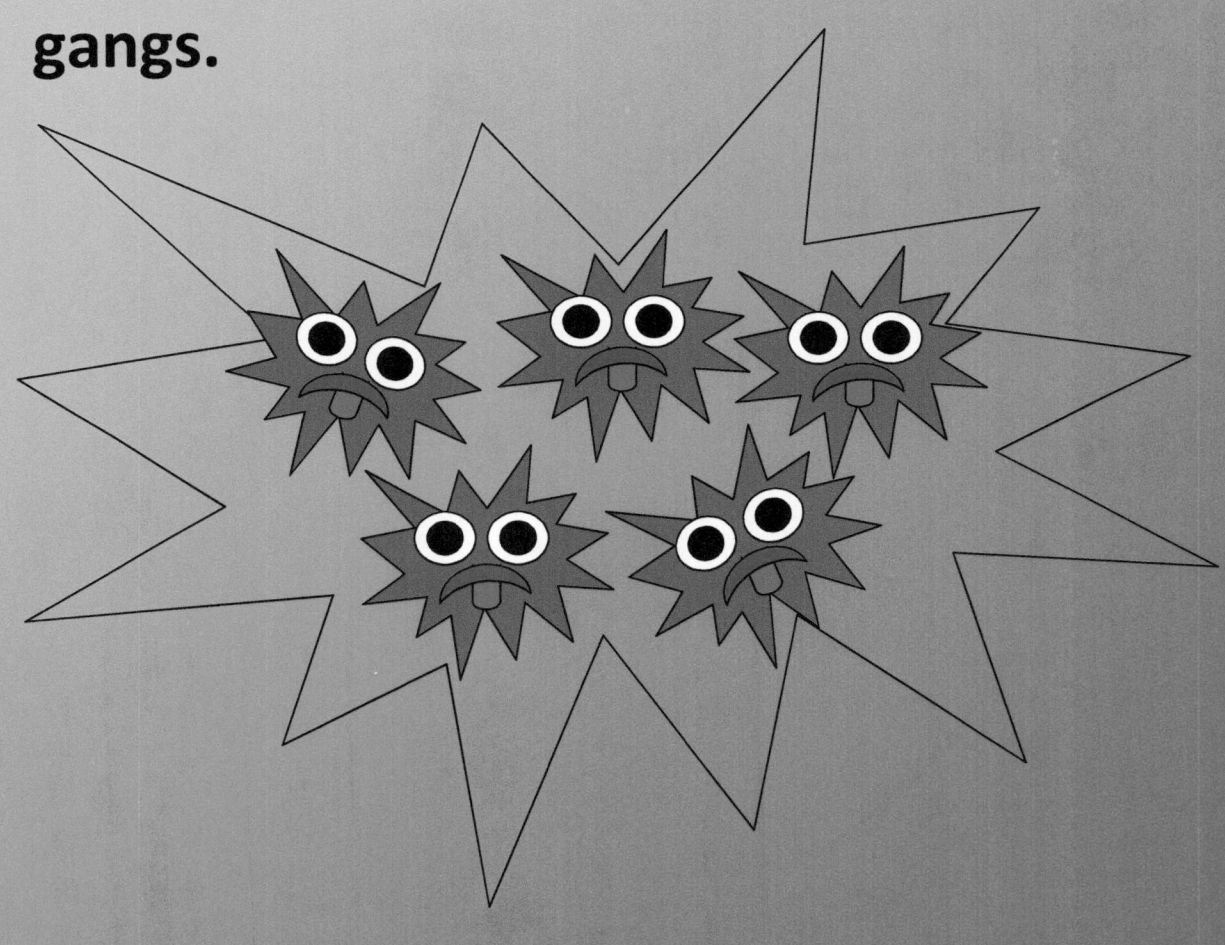

When a gang turns into cancer, the body gets really sick. Soon, the body just gives in to the naughty bad cells. No one can get cancer from another person.

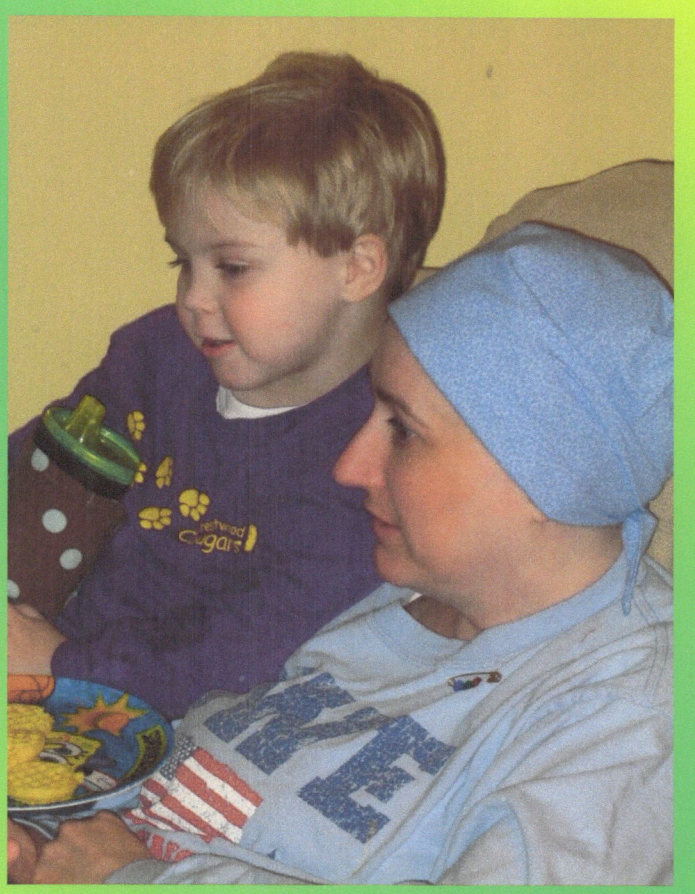

The doctor has to get the naughty gang out of the body.

That way the body can get well and be healthy again.

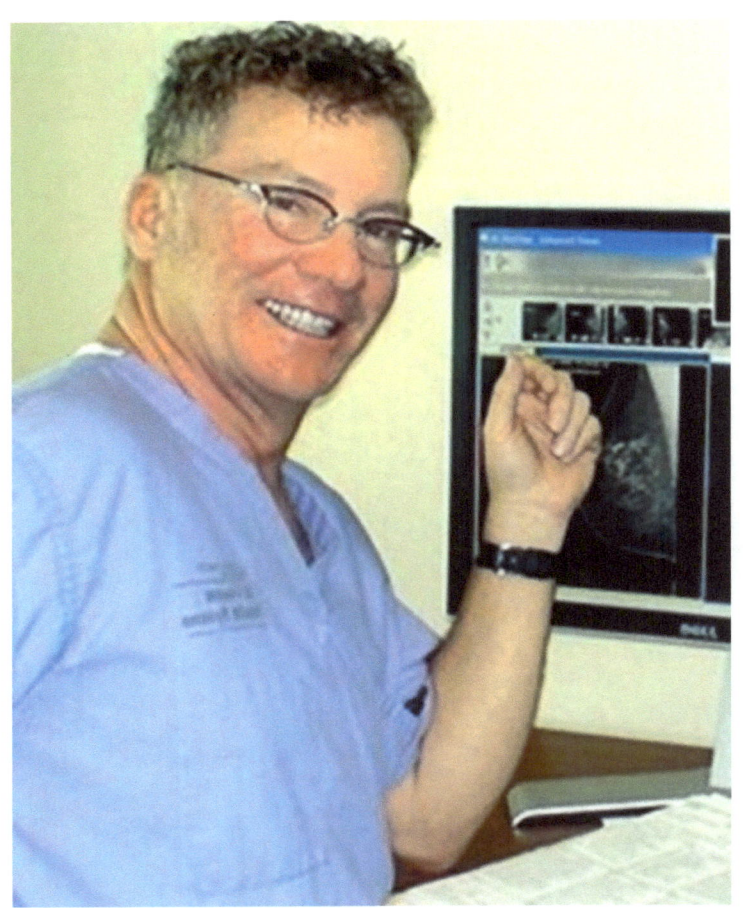

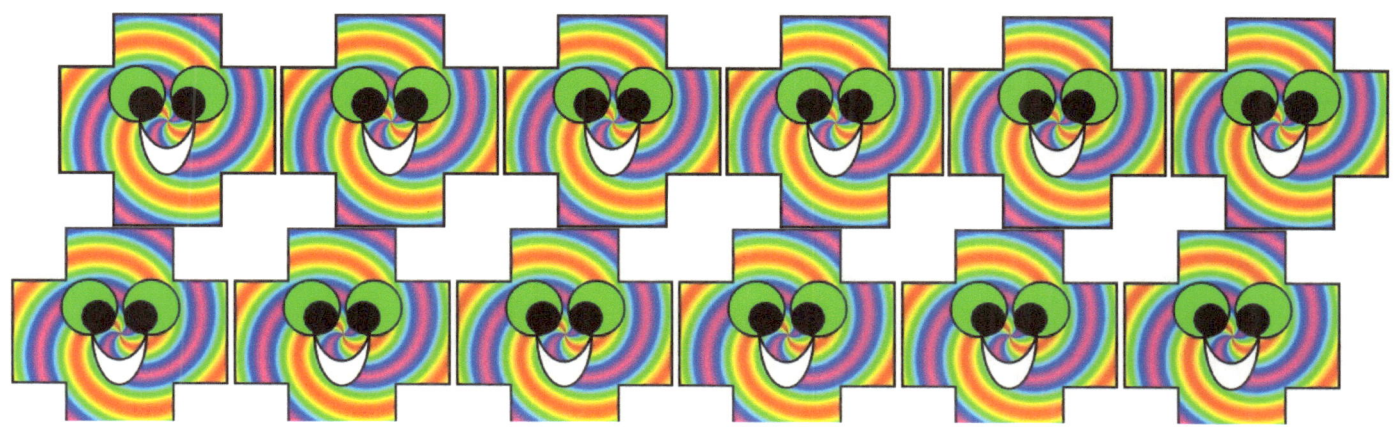

The doctor worries that some bad cells might have been out looking for food or friends when he removed the gang.  Sometimes the doctor decides to send in a group of superheroes called Mighty Cs.  The Mighty Cs are armed with a special medicine… "Chemotherapy". The Mighty Cs go in search of the bad cells.

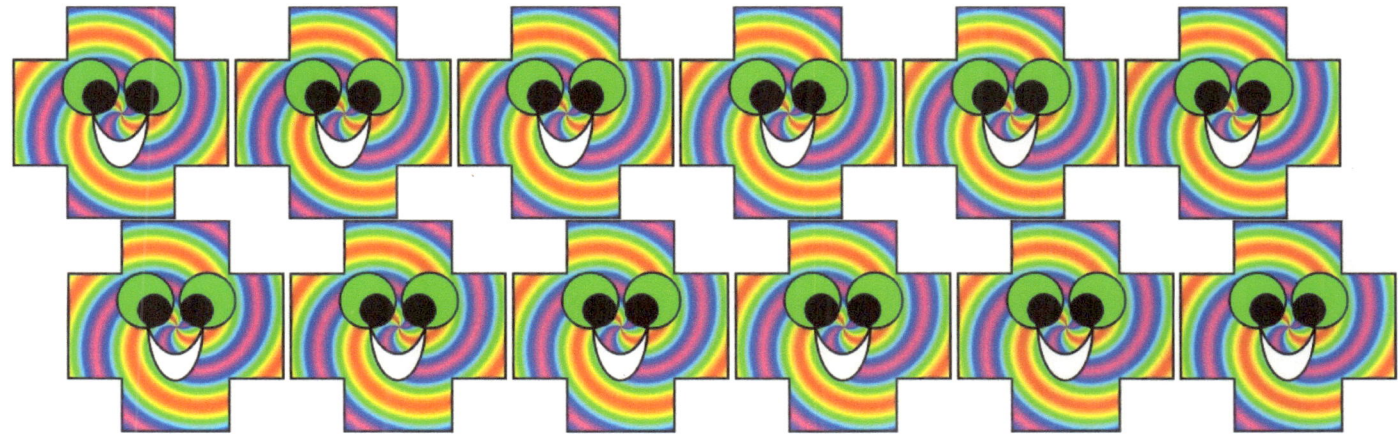

Mighty Cs sometimes get confused and eat some good cells when they are eating the bad cells. This makes the body tired, and sick.

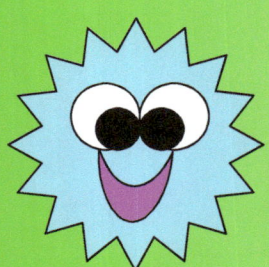

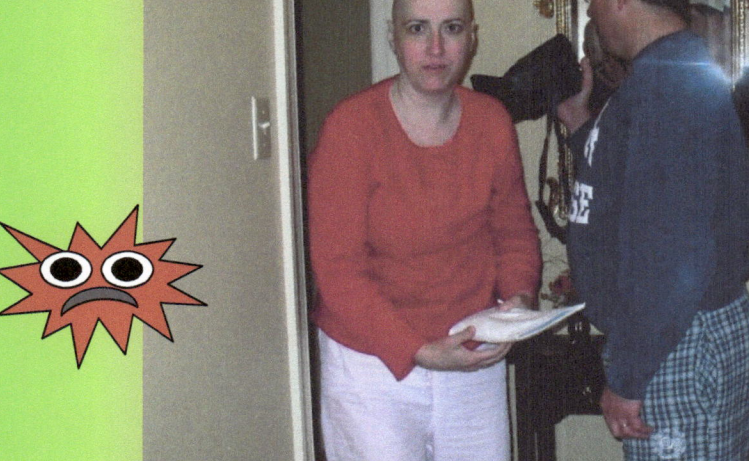

Sometimes the naughty bad cells hold on tight to the hair to try to stay and play in the body. The Mighty Cs push out the hair to get rid of the bad cells.

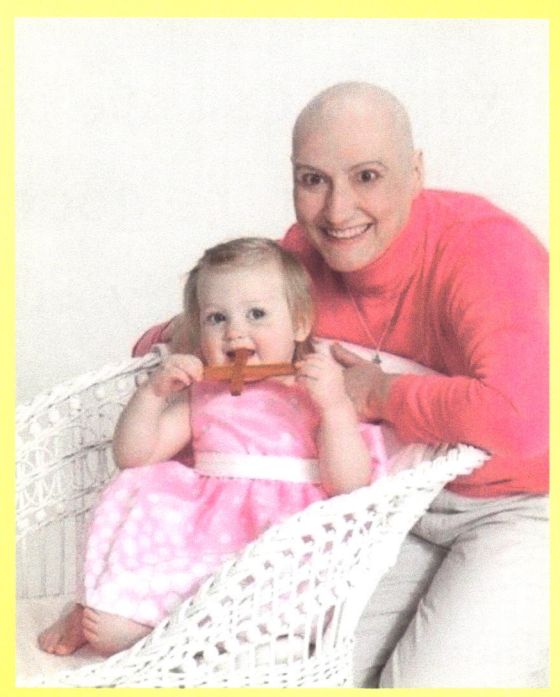

You have to remember that when the hair falls out and the body is tired, the Mighty Cs are trying to win a war and make the body healthy and strong again.

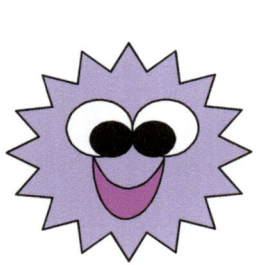
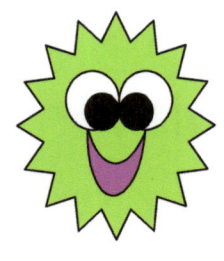
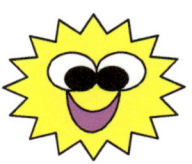
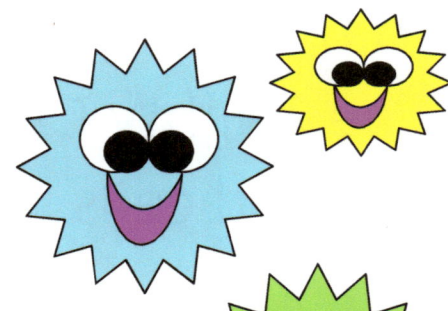

Soon, the Mighty Cs have done their job and all of the good cells take back over the body.  Then, the body begins to become well and happy again.

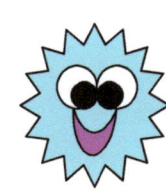

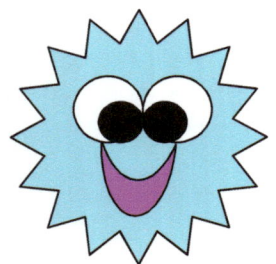

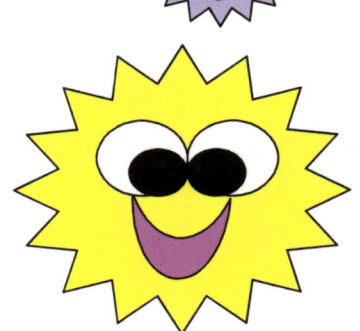
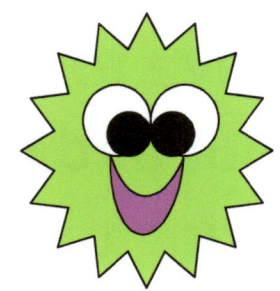

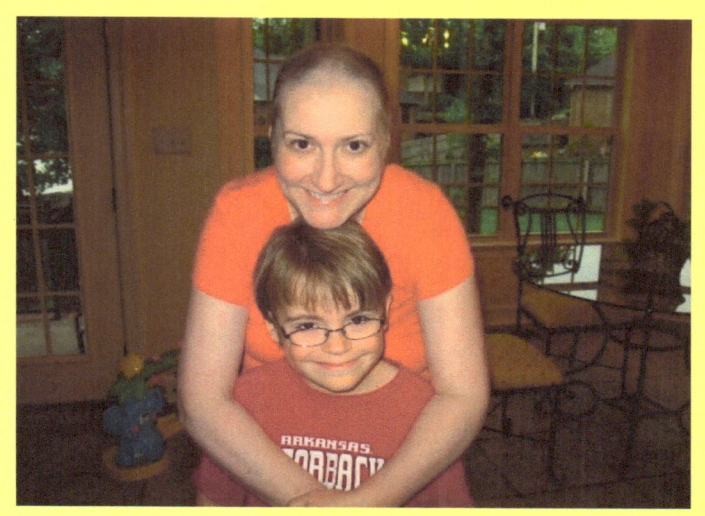 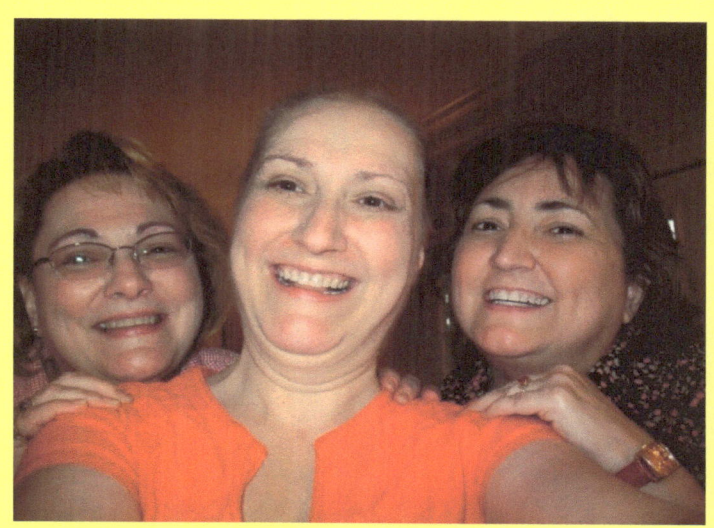

Hair begins to grow!

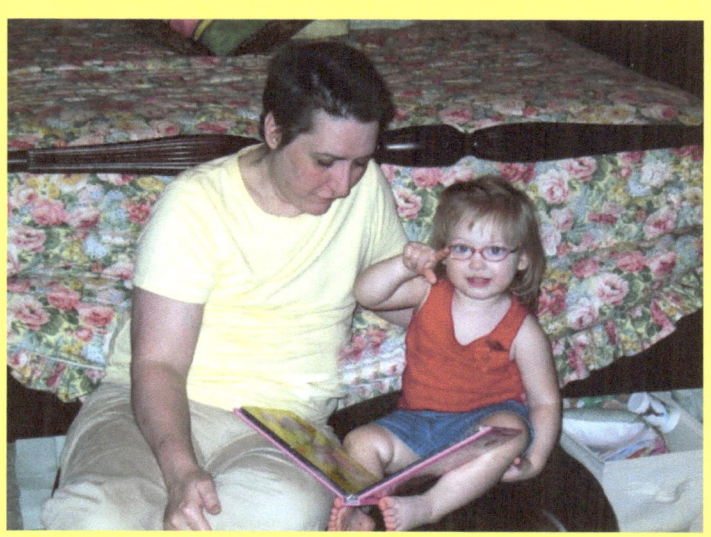

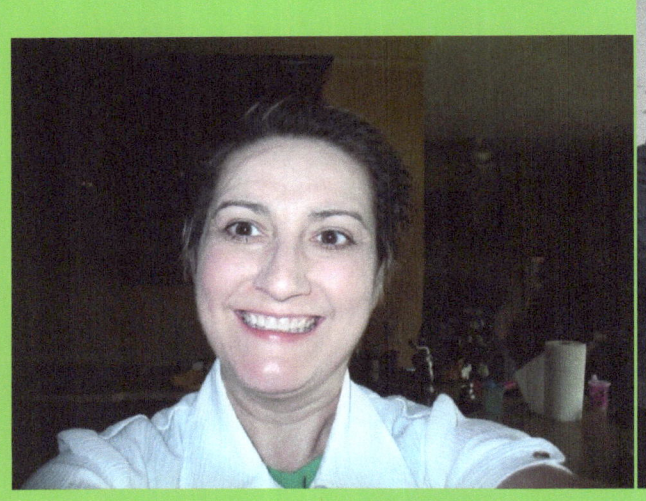

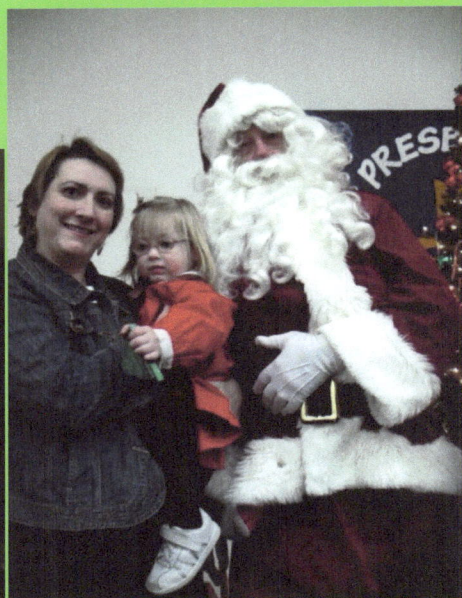

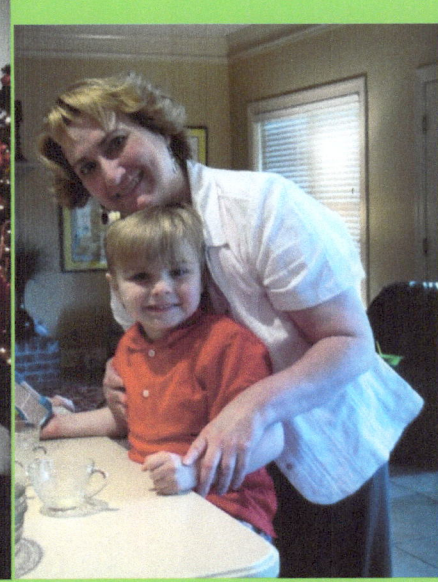

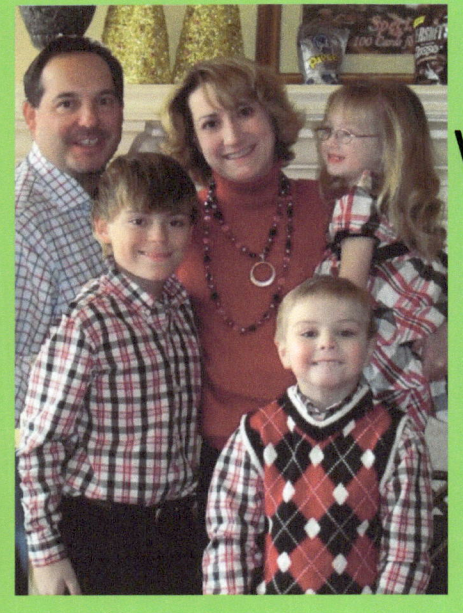

While the hair grows,

the family grows!

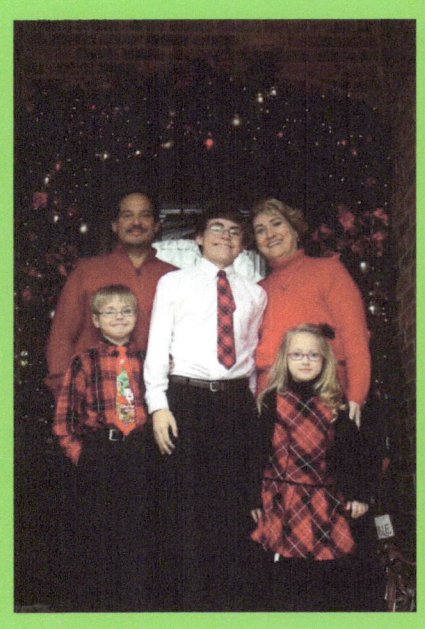

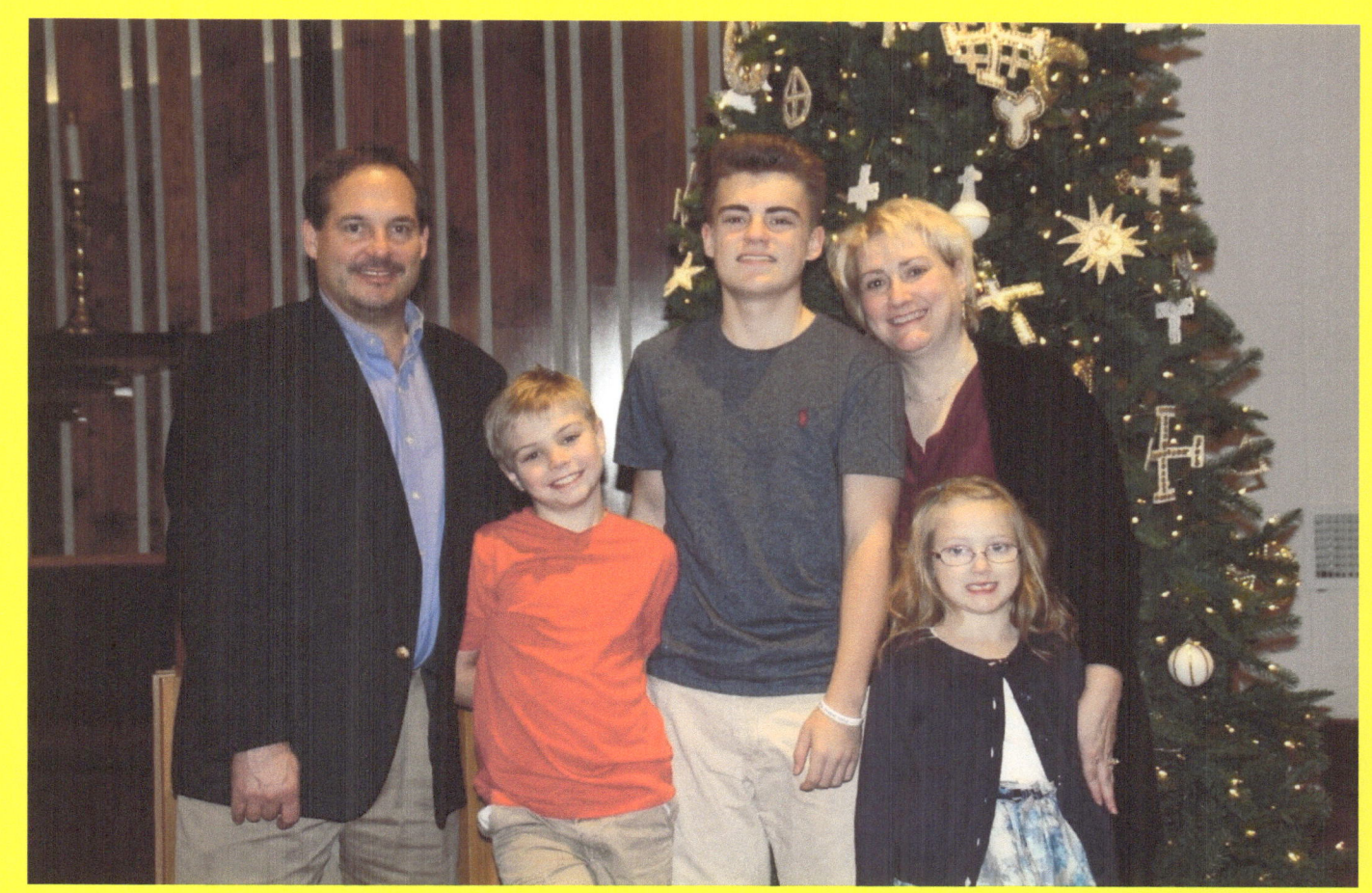

Life is good!

# Add pictures from your journey….

# Mighty C  Vs.  Cancer

Sunny Schellinger Krowski

## ABOUT THE AUTHOR

Sunny Schellinger Krowski born the third girl to her parents Jim and Clarice Schellinger. She has three children but it wasn't until she had her third that she had a girl. Sunny was born and raised in Arkansas and still lives there with her Husband and children. Nine Months after her daughter was born Sunny found a lump while breast feeding. When she found out it was cancer, she wanted to find a way to teach her children about cancer. Sunny loves spending time with her family. She runs several websites for the activities she is active in. Sunny loves being a leader in scouts. She is an active member of Park Hill Presbyterian Church and enjoys the privilege of doing the children's sermon on Sundays.